100 MPH With My Hair On Fire

Bob Benson

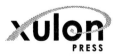

PRESS

Xulon Press
10640 Main Street
Suite 204
Fairfax, VA 22030
(703) 934-4411
XulonPress.com

To order additional copies,
call 1-866-909-BOOK (2665).

Dedication

This book is dedicated to my family, my wife Amy, my two beautiful girls Christie and Anna, the whole Beck clan, Ann, Mike, Michael, Matt, "The Ted Man" and to my parents and Amy's parents, Bette, Bob, Guy and Esther.

A special thank you to my dad. Without him, this book would not have been possible. I thank him for saying yes to the idea and adding his special gifts to this book.

PREFACE

This is a "How To" book. How to have a heart attack before your fortieth birthday. As its author, I speak with some authority. I gave myself one at age thirty-six.

I wrote it for those who are working toward their first coronary; for those few, still living, who have had one but have ignored the signs and symptoms; and for the folks who are struggling through the recovery process. It is also for the loved ones of those people.

This short account of my experience is in response to the interest shown by friends, neighbors and business acquaintances who reluctantly tell me they are also living in a way that makes them candidates for heart problems.

Finally, this is my way of thanking God and all the wonderful people who saved and then changed my life.

CHAPTER 1

In late November, 2000, 59-year-old republican vice presidential nominee, Dick Cheney, suffered a mild heart attack. He was taken to George Washington University medical center where he received an angioplasty procedure. A few days later his doctors told him he could resume his usual schedule and they stressed the importance of good exercise and nutrition. He went on to win the vice presidency. Cheney's reaction to the heart attack was remarkable. He told the media that he had lived with a heart condition for over 20 years but that it did not interfere with his career as a businessman, congressman, defense secretary and White House chief of staff. Actually, it was his fourth heart attack and he had undergone quadruple coronary bypass surgery in 1988. He told the media, "I am unusually blessed."

Actually, Cheney suffered his first heart attack at age 37. It didn't stop him and it didn't make an invalid out of him. Mine came at age 36. The following is the story of how the Lord and I handled my heart attack.

* * * * *

I didn't know it at the time, but there was someone out there who was trying to kill me. With the help of God and a lot of good people, I discovered that the person trying to kill me was me.

Things started to come to a head on October 12, 1996, a fine, crisp Saturday morning. The sun shining through our bedroom window told me the weather would not interfere with the doubles matches set for the morning; so like many other Atlantans I put on my tennis shoes to do battle with some other weekend warriors.

Yeah, a real warrior. I play c-6 tennis. For the unfamiliar let's just say I play bad tennis. In fairness to c-6, what we lack in talent, style and grace, we make up with awkward lunging and frantic slashing of the racket to the tune of Jimmy Connor type grunting. Of particular amusement to the occasional on looker is the manner in which some serve the ball. A disconnected, exaggerated wind-up marked by spastic imbalance that gives false promise of a scorching screamer just over the net, but ends with a sissy sort of slapping motion with the wrist that propels the hapless ball forward with neither pace nor purpose. George Carlin, the famous comedian, says tennis is ping-pong except you get to stand on the table.

I didn't know it then but it is clear to me now that it was that silly game that triggered events that made me grow up, come to grips with the wonders of life and appreciate what caring truly is. More importantly, those events brought with them a calm but certain understanding of what God wants me to know about him and his love. It was the day I stopped running "100 MPH WITH MY HAIR ON FIRE."

I was 36 years old, 6 foot 2, 194 pounds, an OK athlete, nothing special. I truly believed I had the world at my feet. Married to my best friend and the girl of my dreams with two healthy and active daughters in elementary school. Employed by a respected major corporation for 12 years, a top notch benefit package including a new car each year. I traveled the country and the Caribbean visiting beautiful watering holes, meeting sports and entertainment celebrities. I enjoyed first class air travel, the finest accommodations and the best golf courses, all of which I used to sell myself and my employer's products and services. I thought I had it made.

I arrived for the tennis match with my partner, an Englishman. I love the way he talks with that clipped accent that gives him an aura of dignity and authority.

"Good show mate, splendid shot," he offered as my backhand accidentally landed in bounds. I remember thinking that if I could borrow that accent, people would have to be impressed.

We warmed up with our opponents in the cool of the morning and exchanged the pleasantries typical of the neighborhood tennis venue. The match began fairly well as we won the first set. We dropped the second by a whisker and got ready for the third and final set. My partner and I went to the bench for a quick cold drink and a fast wipe of the face with a towel.

"You are puffing rather laboriously," noted my English companion.

"Yeah, I must really be out of shape. I have to do something about it," I said without an ounce of sincerity.

We both laughed and returned to the court for the final set, which started on a positive note but unraveled at the end, and we lost. No big deal. Better luck next week. We shook hands with the victors and walked to the commons area for something to eat and to review the highs and lows with friends that had gathered to watch.

During the 30-minute chit chat session, I inhaled a couple of hot dogs and washed them down with two cans of Coke.

"I have to get home and cut the grass," I said to the

group. "We're having a cookout in the backyard tonight with some folks and I'm sure Amy (my beautiful wife) has a list of stuff I have to get to before the guests show up. Sorry you guys can't come but it's for ritzy people only."

"Oh, then you'll be wearing shoes for a change," said my English partner. You have to love that British humor!

I jumped in my car and drove the quarter- mile back to the house, stopping at the mailbox. As I reached for the mail, it happened. I didn't know it then, but what was about to transpire changed me and a whole lot of other folks, too. God touched me not so gently and quietly told me, "You're running a little too hot, it's time to slow down and find out what this world is really about." Those might not have been his exact words because the message didn't come over some celestial loudspeaker. It came into my mind very clearly, however, and make no mistake, that was the message and He was the messenger!

I know I may be starting to lose some of you. Another religious wacko who thinks he converses with God. Let me explain my position. It's not very complicated. I don't think something can be true and untrue at the same time. Therefore, either there is a God or there isn't. As adults we have to make choices. We are free to believe in God or we can believe there is no God. There is no scientific proof either way. We can also shrug our shoulders and take the position that we just don't know one way or the other. Those are the folks who pray, "Dear God, if there is one, save my soul if I have one." I'm not the brightest person in the world but I know I have plenty of company in believing that there is a God. I think it's called faith. I also have decided that God is not aloof and incommunicado but rather is a loving God who communicates with mortals. Again, to me that's a no brainer. I got one of His messages.

CHAPTER 2

As I closed the mailbox, there was a tight discomfort in my chest. It was not debilitating but I was certainly feeling a feeling that I had never felt before.

"What the heck is that?," I asked myself aloud.

My first hope was that I was having some exotic form of heartburn brought on by the two-hot-dog-and-Coke combination. I guess I knew I was kidding myself but I wasn't ready to face any other options.

I pulled the car up the driveway and into the garage, got out and climbed the four steps to the kitchen entry door. Amy was in the kitchen preparing things for the party. She smiled and asked how the tennis match turned out and reminded me the lawn needed mowing. She saw nothing in my appearance to suggest I was having a physical problem because there was nothing to see. I sat down at the kitchen table and told her of the discomfort in my chest and that it now felt like I had metal bands around my elbows that were tight and somewhat uncomfortable.

"Amy, something's wrong."

She saw I wasn't playing games. "What do you think it is?"

"Something does not feel right here in the middle of my chest," I said, as I gently tapped above my sternum.

"Maybe it's something you ate." She knew me and my devotion to frankfurters.

"Yeah, maybe," I answered as I got up to go upstairs to lie down. I went to the bedroom closet and grabbed an old blood pressure monitor that I had picked up while at college. During a routine physical at the end of my senior year at East Carolina University they discovered a borderline blood pressure elevation and put me on a baby dose of a beta-blocker. Beta-blockers act to block every day stresses from triggering a rise in blood pressure. I chalked it all up to too many beers and too many parties. I bought the blood pressure monitor to make sure the pills worked their magic. My pressure returned to normal within that year.

I laid down on the bed and took my blood pressure. Obviously, I knew what I was looking for and

I feared what was going on inside me. I was afraid and didn't want to face it. I wanted to be able to laugh later and tell people that those damn hot-dogs did such a job on me that I thought I was having a heart attack. My hopes picked up a little when I saw that my pressure was 140 over 90. That's only borderline and I had imagined it would be going through the roof.

I laid there flat on my back flapping my arms like a chicken trying to chase away the tightness around my elbows. Picture Mick Jagger at a concert with a thumb under each armpit flapping his elbows up and down. That was me trying to feel normal.

"Oh God, please let me feel normal." And in an instant, my prayer was answered. The odd feelings that had come over me lasted a total of a little over a fifteen minutes and then they were gone. There was never any real pain and I was never doubled over from any of the sensations I felt. I thought I could just go about my business as usual, but that's not quite what God had in mind.

I think everyone vaguely anticipates the possibility of a heart attack and, for that reason, people ask me to explain the feelings I had that morning so they will know what it is if it comes. I understand, however, that symptoms vary greatly depending on the exact problem and the individual involved. I can only tell you how I felt: Picture yourself in a dentist chair as they are about to x-ray your teeth. On goes a kind of lead blanket to protect the rest of your body from the x-rays. Now take two of those blankets, fold them in 8-inch squares and lay them one on top of the other in the center of your chest between your nipples. Then take a pair of handcuffs and place one around each elbow, and tighten them down until they are cutting off the circulation-but not so tight that they actually cause you pain. Finally, have someone scare the pants off you and there you have it.

CHAPTER 3

I came back downstairs and found Amy phoning around the neighborhood to some of our neighbors who are nurses to see if they might shed some light on my weird feelings. Amy reported that the rough consensus seemed to be indigestion.

"I'm with them," I said with a nagging lack of conviction.

Then the phone rang and it was our neighbor across the street. She was the first person Amy had called, but there had been no answer. (I'm not using real names in much of this account in order to avoid any possible embarrassment. I'll call my neighbor "Angela" because she was one of the primary *angels* that God assigned to my case.)

Angela called to find out if we needed to borrow their lawn mower. She and her husband were to be guests at our cookout and I had mentioned to her that I needed to borrow a mower because mine was out of service. Angela is a physician's assistant. Amy told her my symptoms and Angela asked to speak with me. It turned out that Angela also had a solid background in cardiac cases.

"How are you doing?"

"A little tired but fine. No more pressure or bands around my elbows."

"Can you make those feelings come back?"

"Angela, the last thing in the world I want to do is make those feelings come back," I said.

Angela kept boring in. "Yes, I know, but I want you to push on the places that you had the discomfort and see if you can bring the feelings back."

She explained that if I had strained something playing tennis I would be able to feel the sensations over and over by massaging the affected muscles.

After some prodding and kneading, I reported that I was unable to recreate the sensations that had hit me at the mailbox.

"Go to St. Joseph's hospital now and get yourself checked out," she ordered.

"No way, Angela. I really feel fine and I'd feel silly going to the hospital. It was the hotdogs and it's gone now."

"Just get it checked out Bob. It may take a couple of hours but they can ease your mind about what you were feeling."

I thanked her and hung up the phone. Angela knew exactly what was happening to me. She didn't tell me then but she called it right on the money. I found that out later from her husband. An important point to be made here is that most men and perhaps women who have, had or will experience the sensations that I did will/would/may blow them off as nothing. Listen real carefully here, if I had blown off these sensations as nothing, I probably would be DEAD right now. Do not blow off strange sensations you feel, your body is trying to tell you something. I beg of you to listen to your body.

CHAPTER 4

J ack Nicholson played a grizzled Marine colonel in the movie, "A Few Good Men". In a dramatic scene, he sat in the witness box in a court-martial under blistering cross examination by Tom Cruise, who played a young JAG lawyer. The lawyer heatedly demanded the truth from the colonel and the colonel snarled back at him, "YOU CAN'T HANDLE THE TRUTH."

Handling the truth is sometimes very difficult. The tough first step is to face it. When you are 36 years old, handling news of your own heart attack can be a bit of a chore.

My Dad gave me a ride to St. Joseph's, one of the finest cardiac care facilities in the U.S. My parents live between our house and the hospital. Coincidence that my parents live in Atlanta and so do I? A guy born in Pennsylvania, lived most of his childhood in New Jersey went to school in the Carolinas, works in the Carolinas while his parents live in New Jersey. His parents get transferred to Atlanta from New Jersey and then I do to three years later. I don't think so, God sets this stuff up way in advance.

Christie, our eldest daughter, was out in the boondocks at a horse farm and would be stranded unless someone went to pick her up. Amy knew the way to the horse farm and Dad didn't. Dad had been to St. Joseph's before and Amy hadn't, so Dad got the driving assignment. Later, Amy regretted not taking me but, at the time, she knew I was in good hands and that time was of the essence.

Dad and I pulled up at the door to St. Joseph's emergency room. I got out and walked in like I was picking up a half-gallon of milk at the grocery store. I felt kind of silly, no rolling in on a gurney with interns pounding on my chest, just strolled in like I was visiting a sick friend.

Dad parked the car and then joined me in the waiting room. By that time, I had signed in and given up my insurance card, name, address and other requested information and was told I would be seen by the triage nurse. Most medical terms come from the Greek and many military terms come from the French. "Triage" is a French military term that actually means "sorting." It is the sorting of casualties of war to determine the sequence and place of treatment.

By then it was still early afternoon so the emergency room was pretty quiet. Later, some of the victims of Atlanta's Saturday night madness would begin to show up and the place would be jumping.

Time passed very slowly in that waiting room, but before long we were joined by the triage nurse. She looked at a gentleman across from us and asked him his problem and his age.

"I have pain in my chest and I'm 56," he said without raising his head.

She looked at me. "How about you?"

"I had some chest pressure earlier today and a funny feeling around my elbows. It's gone now and I'm 36."

She quickly grabbed the other guy and away they went. I felt like I had been rejected at an audition for a part I didn't want. Dad and I laughed and agreed it must have been my age and robust appearance. I started to believe that going there had been a waste of time.

After about 20 minutes the triage nurse returned and took me to have my vital signs checked. I gave her a run-down of what had happened. I told her I wanted to make sure it wasn't a heart attack.

"You are too young to have a heart attack. It was probably the hotdogs," she laughed.

I really liked that lady! "So I can go home now?,"

I asked while making motions as if to leave. She caught me half out of the seat and explained that the rules called for me to see a doctor. She took me to another room, had me lie down and hooked me up to a heart monitor.

"The doctor will be with you soon," she said as she headed for the door. She must have told my father where I was because he came in and sat next to my bed. What did she mean by "soon" we kept asking each other as we waited? Dad said we probably took the word out of context and that she meant it to mean something like, "World War II followed 'soon' after World War I."

CHAPTER 5

As we waited, Dad divided his time among telling me dopey jokes to keep my spirits up and calling Amy to give her a blow by blow. He kept telling her that if she came to the hospital as she wanted to, I would probably be sent home before she got here. In between phone calls to Amy, Dad kept running out to the reception room to check the score of the Notre Dame-Navy game on TV. South Bend is Mecca to Dad. Another thing you want to remember: love your parents with all your heart. It's real simple, if not for them, there is no you. Love your parents!

Finally, a doctor who was about my age showed up, heard my story, listened to my heart, learned I didn't smoke and cast another preliminary vote for the hotdogs theory. Again, I could smell the front door.

Then the young doctor started pulling on his chin with the tips of his fingers as he pondered setting me free. "I'm probably being overly cautious but let's take an EKG," he said, dashing out of the room. Within minutes, in came a technician rolling a machine and proceeded to hook fifteen electrodes to my body and some sort of clip to my finger, and then started the machine. The electrocardiogram listens to the beat of the heart and traces the series of beats with a pen on a long strip of paper. It takes no more than two minutes and there is no pain or discomfort involved in the procedure. Doctors can read those wavy lines produced by the EKG and learn a bundle about what's going on with the heart.

The technician whisked the machine out of the room and almost immediately the young doctor came back peering at the EKG tape and pulling on his chin with his fingers again.

"This looks normal," he said as my spirits soared.

"Great," I replied.

"But there is this little squiggle here," he said as he showed me a down stroke on the tape that was just the slightest bit different than the hundreds of other scratches on the paper.

"We have also tested your blood to see if there has been an elevation of an enzyme that is triggered by a heart problem."

"How did I make out on that test?"

"There was no sign of an enzyme elevation."

"Great," I repeated.

He stared into the corner for a few seconds then he asked me if I had ever had an EKG before and, if so, whether anyone had mention the little squiggle. I answered "yes" to his first question and "no" to his second.

"Hmmm," he said.

"Hey Doc. Doesn't the blood test result fortify the hotdog theory?" I'm pushing the guy to parole me but he's going to make up his own professional mind. God bless him for that!

"Sometimes it takes that enzyme twenty four hours to show up. I may be wasting your time but I want a cardiologist to look at you."

"How long will that take?"

"Dr. Margolis is on duty. He should be able to see you soon."

That word "soon" again. Dad called Amy, handed me the phone and went out again to check the Notre Dame score. I brought Amy up to date and I could hear in her voice that she thought things were dragging on too long and that the hot-dog theory might be coming apart. I told her the theory was still the front runner but these medical people like to be cautious. I told her that I still thought I would be sent home. I told her I loved her and that I would see her shortly.

Dad came back. The Irish won a squeaker. We took up waiting again. Since neither of us had ever seen Dr. Margolis, we each described how we thought he would look when he finally appeared and we made a gentlemen's bet as to who would come the closest. I think Dad won but events quickly drew my mind to other things.

CHAPTER 6

Doctor Margolis decided to keep me overnight. He seemed to read from the same script as the others. It was probably nothing and, 'sorry to put you through the inconvenience but you are here now so let's keep you over just to be safe.'

I had never spent a night in a hospital and I felt fine. I had pumped myself up for a night back in my own bed with Amy, and with Anna and Christie in their rooms down the hall. Doctor Margolis agreed I was too young for a heart attack and that there had been no test results indicating otherwise.

In frustration, I looked at Dad. His face seemed to say, "I know how you feel but you have no choice. You stay."

I turned to Doctor Margolis and looked him in the eye. "If it were you, would you stay over?"

His response was firm but kindly, "Of course."

My emotional roller coaster was on another down-slope and I started to do some first rate worrying. "Why me? Why now? What next?" I kept clinging to the fact that none of these experts had told me I had a heart attack. At the same time, all of them were allowing for the slim possibility that I did. I felt like a guy in California after an earthquake waiting for the next tremor or the next big one.

If it was a heart attack, what kind was it? The kind that winds up killing you? The kind that turns the man of the house into some feeble wreck that eventually gets on everyone's nerves?

I hadn't had enough adversity in my life to toughen me up for this sort of thing. I didn't know if I could handle the truth if it was the kind of bad news I was beginning to anticipate.

This was my heart they were talking about, not some ancillary organ. The heart of the matter. I love you with all my heart. Have a heart. You broke my heart. Serious as a heart attack. This was the muscle I was counting on to provide me with a long long life. I was one scared puppy.

Another call to Amy and she hurried to the hospital with the kids who brought me hastily homemade get well cards that told me they loved me. By that time I was in a private room and had sampled the gourmet delights from the kitchen. The chef was of the "hospital bland" school.

Anna, our youngest, was eight years old at the time and I could see she was frightened by the fact that I was in bed with tubes and monitors hooked up to me. I tried to be upbeat with her but she was having her own battle handling the truth. The hospital was an alien place to her and she didn't want me in there. She had seen enough television to know that people died in hospitals. I also think she saw them sticking me with a needle and, to her, that was terrifying.

After they left, I spent a fitful night worrying over what news the morning would bring. I also had a monitor on me that continuously observed the beat of my heart and every two hours or so some angel of mercy would drop by to shove in another needle and sample my blood. It got to the point where I hardly woke up for the prick of the needle.

I did a lot of praying and it came to me that lately all my prayers had been of the, "Gimme, Get me, Save me, Let me," variety. God hadn't heard many, "Thank you" type prayers from me. I wondered how it would be to try to keep a friend if every time I spoke to him, it was to ask a favor. I decided then that I should change my prayer habits. I should pray for others not myself. I should offer up my random acts of kindness as a plea for others in need. As for me and my future, "Thy Will Be Done". I said that to myself but I knew I needed to work on it.

CHAPTER 7

Sunday ranks as one of the worst and best days of my life all wrapped up in one. I awoke early and my parents soon arrived with their thermos of coffee. My mom went through all the mother questions. "Did you eat yet? Did you sleep well? How are you feeling? Would you like me to fix your pillow?"

Amy arrived with Christie, our eldest. Anna had begged off coming to the hospital and I understood fully.

Doctor Margolis made his rounds early on Sunday; he was at my door with a knock. I tried to look into his eyes to see if I could read what the news was before he said anything. I'm pretty good at reading people but his face gave away nothing. He didn't make us wait long for the news. With Mom and Dad, Amy and Christie by my side, he said: "Well we were right."

For a millisecond I was filled with joy! "We were right!" The wiener theory had prevailed! This 36-year-old has not had a heart attack!

But then, of course he finished the sentence. "I'm keeping you overnight because you have had a HEART ATTACK." I was lying on the hospital bed with Christie's hand in mine. It's a wonder she didn't yelp the way I squeezed it.

Doctor Margolis went on to explain that the results of the blood work taken throughout the night clearly showed the telltale elevation of enzyme levels in my blood stream, a sure sign of a heart attack. Known in the medical world as a Myocardial Infarction, the attack is caused by the blockage of an artery that shuts down the normal blood flow to the heart. Many things can cause that blockage.

In his best bedside manner, Dr. Margolis said it was probably a minor attack and it was most likely some artery in the back of the heart or one so small that they may not be able to find anything at all. He didn't say so but I think he guessed it was a mild attack because I was still there, alive and listening to him. He went on to explain that they would probably want to do an angiogram to further diagnose the problem.

We quizzed him about the procedure and whether he would be performing it. Dr. Margolis explained that he and his doctor partners worked as a team and that he didn't handle the invasive procedures. He assured us that his partners had all done hundreds of angiograms and they were all board certified and well qualified. The more I listened to Dr. Margolis, the more I liked him. Kind, caring and very, very, competent. Later, Dad told me he felt the same way but to be safe, he called another doctor, a close friend, for a run down on the Margolis team. The word came back that I couldn't be in better hands.

The procedure was set for Monday, the next morning. I was to relax and watch some of the in-house videos on the procedure. Relax? Better said than done. Let's see, I've got a wife, two young kids, a mortgage, two educations to take care of, and if I'm lucky, two weddings (and only two) to attend, walk down the aisle and pay for. Then I've got grandchildren to give sage and wise advice to and to brag about until I bore listeners to tears. What will my heart attack do to those plans?

In the near term, I've got to be in Tahoe on Wednesday and in Miami on Friday. Work is tremendously busy and stressful due to the continuous internal changes being made and quotas to meet. The company wants me to move to Chicago, but they won't give me a date nor will they commit to a time frame. There are budget problems, personnel problems, internal politics problems, and I'm convinced that none of them can be solved without yours truly. I was thinking of that country song, "Lord this time you gave me a mountain. You gave me a mountain to climb."

Yep, time to relax, Bob, and watch the videos. Somehow I did. Not relax, I watched the videos.

Amy and I became closer that Sunday. We thought we were truly one before, but that Sunday we became an even better team and our love deepened. Facing that kind of crisis can make or break you as a couple. It never leaves you the same as you were before. I had married a trooper and she was everything I needed her to be. In sickness and in health. They were not empty words.

There were a lot of moist eyes that day. A lot of soul searching and unasked questions about God's reason for selecting me for this challenge. My Mom was upset but doing her best not to show it. Dad, who never cries-that is, his expression doesn't change-was just staring out the window, probably talking with God trying to figure it all out. He never cries but in an emotional situation his eyes tear to the point that water starts dripping off his chin. I know how he felt. This whole thing was backwards. A 64-year-old man staring out the window of his 36 year old son's hospital room thinking about his son's heart attack. I know how I'd feel if one of my kids was seriously hurt. I'd want to take their place but I'd be helpless to do so. It was just a very emotional time. Why was all this happening? I'm convinced there was a good reason. Wondrous as it is, the human mind has its limitations. Consequently, trying to understand God, who is infinite in His wisdom, is like trying to empty the ocean into a tea cup. God works in mysterious ways but if you keep your mind and heart (no pun intended) open to Him and listen, He will speak to you. There was a reason for my being on my back in that hospital, I just needed to pray and figure it out. I would understand in His time.

A priest came to my door. He had noticed on my registration that I was a Catholic and he asked if Amy and I wanted to receive communion. I jumped at the chance because I wanted to be as close to God as I could get.

Imagine that you're a kid walking home alone from school and you turn a corner and walk right into the town bully, a real thug who's too big for his age and takes great joy in taking the likes of you apart and stomping on the pieces. Terror sets in. Now imagine the same scene but this time you are not alone. Your big brother is with you. Your big brother, who is kind and gentle but even the bully knows he is not to be messed with. This time no terror, no fear, no problem.

I wanted God to be with me when I turned that corner tomorrow. The priest opened his case to distribute communion and he put a purple vestment around my neck. I was a little taken aback by this as most times when you see this type of thing on TV or in the movies it was what we Catholics call "the last rites." The last rites always meant that death was hovering nearby. It was a sacrament that was a kind of a final send off, the last thing they did before they pulled the sheet up over your head and turned out the lights. When I asked the good padre if he was sure he was in the right room, he assured me that this was the prayer of the sick and was not the last rites. Amy and I chuckled nervously and went on to receive communion.

The same priest came by everyday of my stay and had communion for me. It was very peaceful and I looked forward to his visits.

CHAPTER 8

*A*my and my parents spent most of the day with me and in the evening Amy, Christie and Anna, who overcame her fears, returned. Hospitals are boring for kids but I'll tell you my kids came and stayed as long as they could stand it because they knew their Dad needed them. I didn't have to ask, they just knew somehow. They choked me up good when they handed me "Muttsy" and "Squeaky Baby". Most kids, and mine are no exception, have stuffed toys they take to bed every night. I don't how many times Amy and I had to scour the house looking for either Muttsy or Squeaky Baby because the kids' going to bed was unthinkable without them. Now, here they were, giving up their security by lending me these well-worn friends to help me get through the night.

That's real sacrifice folks and it's family. There

was no corporation, bank account, government, possession, diploma, mansion or stock portfolio sitting around my bed that Sunday. It was my family, the sustaining unit of love. I was thinking about that and about reordering my priorities.

Sunday, as I mentioned earlier, was video day. I was to watch on the in house video programming the angiogram and angioplasty procedure "Angio" is the Greek word for blood vessel. The angiogram procedure is an exploratory procedure, used to see where, and what arteries are blocked. It involves the insertion of a dye into the arteries and the use of x-ray. Angioplasty, on the other hand, is the procedure they use to actually clear the blockage if they can get to it without opening your chest.

Why couldn't I be in front of my own TV in my own home watching a movie we just rented from Blockbuster? Noooooo! I had to watch Angio movies! Amy and I watched the videos alone. Mom and Dad took the girls for some lunch and Amy and I got out the pamphlets and the remote control and cranked up some videos. We were to watch the procedural videos and then sign a document releasing all involved from any responsibility should something bad happen during the procedure. It was no light entertainment. With all the malpractice cases that hospitals and doctors face, they have come up with procedures to make sure patients know the details of any treatment in advance so that consent is given will full knowledge. They make sure the patient is aware of possible complications and risk. Of course, one risk includes dying on the operating table! We watched as the video explained all of what happens from start to finish. We cried a little, we cried some more, we hugged awhile, said a few prayers and then signed the documents.

It was right about then that Amy and I started talking about selling the house, buying a smaller, less expensive place with no mortgage, moving to the beach and fishing off some dock for the rest of our lives. We had to get out of the rat race. We didn't need this extremely fast pace in our lives. It was literally killing me.

I reviewed with Amy our assets and accounts; where the will was and the steps we were taking to provide for the girls' educations. Insurance policies were paid up if, God forbid, anything went wrong; she and the kids would have something to go on. Talk about a tough conversation to have with your best friend! Amy told me to stop talking like that because everything would be fine. We held hands, sobbed and just sat there thinking the rest of the day.

Hal Roach, the Irish comedian, tells a story that fit my situation. It seems that Father Kelly was walking back to the rectory very late at night after visiting a sick parishioner. As he passed Murphy's pub, he heard laughter and singing so he knew that some of the lads were still in there drinking up their pay. Father Kelly burst through the door and yelled, "If any of you heathens want to go to heaven raise your hands."

All of the hands shot up except Flanagan's and he just kept staring into his pint of Guinness.

"Mike Flanagan, do you mean to stand there and tell me that someday you don't want to go to heaven?," thundered Father Kelly.

" Oh someday, sure Father. I thought you were leaving right now."

During the day, I had a call from my sister Ann, who lives with her husband Mike and three sons in Cherry Hill, New Jersey. She gave me a pep talk, told me she loved me and would keep me in her prayers. We did our best to make each other laugh.

Late Sunday evening, everyone had gone home. Amy really wanted to stay at the hospital with me but we both knew the kids needed her. They had to be readied for school the next morning. As I prepared for sleep Sunday night a nurse came in, studied her clipboard and told me I was scheduled to be first in the morning for the catheter lab where the angios are performed. I was asked if I would like a sleeping pill to help me rest. Something told me to decline, which I did.

Part of my job involves giving presentations at

high level meetings or to large groups. Often these are high pressure situations in which I stand open to challenge by subordinates, peers, bosses and various levels of brass. Normally, the night before such a presentation I would toss and turn, going over the materials in my head and trying to anticipate the questions that were sure to fly my way. I would barely get any rest.

So I was figuring that I was in for a long night. This was going to be a pretty important meeting. It had to go right but I had no control. There would be no point during the night when I would feel prepared for this one and the stakes were tremendous.

I closed my eyes and slept like a baby. God was with me every REM sleep of the way. It's hard to explain but, man, what a good feeling. I wasn't worried. I wasn't anxious. God was with me. I was certain I could trust in Him and He wouldn't let me down. I felt His presence. It was going to be okay. Trust in God is a powerful thing. Without it is to be a rudderless boat in a hurricane. When you live and breathe this trust, your entire being becomes content and satisfied. I was ready to turn the corner and look who I had with me!

CHAPTER 9

Monday morning I was up early, brushed my teeth, washed my face. I was ready man. Bring on the Catheter lab. Mom and Dad showed up around 7:15. Again they had their coffee thermos with them but they looked as if they hadn't slept as well as I had. Amy arrived a little after Mom and Dad. She had that fear of the unknown in her eyes but was trying her best not to show it.

The shuttle guy, (the guy who took me down to the lab in the wheel chair) showed up right on time for the trip. I had on one of those terrible gowns, open in the back and nothing underneath it. The shuttle guy covered me good with blankets so the people we passed in the hall wouldn't be treated to a view of my bum. I also wore my NY Yankees base-ball hat. A bit of bravado calculated to show the world that I was without fear. You may recall the Yankees were to play the hometown Atlanta Braves that October in the World Series.

Amy, Mom and Dad followed behind, joined us on the elevator and then followed again until we reached a set of swinging doors. The shuttle guy smiled at them and said, "Here's where we leave you folks. Time for hugs and kisses and then you may wait in the family waiting room. You'll be kept posted on how Joe DiMaggio here is doing."

I got my hugs and kisses, we said our goodbyes and our see ya' soons. The shuttle guy pushed me through the swinging doors then left me in the hall for a while as they prepared the lab and waited for the lab team to arrive. Silently, I was giving them all a pep talk. "I hope you all had plenty of sleep folks because we need perfection in the lab today. No errors or strike-outs."

A few young nurses and doctors walked by and made fun of the Yankees cap. Someone said I was too young to be there. I know, I know already. They asked if I smoked and whether my condition was hereditary. They should have asked if I had been running 100 MPH with my hair on fire!

Finally, I got rolled into the lab. My first impression was how icy cold it was. The video said it would be. The apparatus in there needs a cool environment to work effectively. If that's the case, let it snow for all I care! A nice nurse had covered my bare toes in the hall, she must have known about the arctic chill.

They eased me out of the chair and up onto the table in the middle of a large room. There were monitors and gadgets everywhere. The videos were starting to payoff as I recognized a lot of the stuff.

For the procedure, you have your inner upper thigh shaved on both sides. They gave me a choice so I opted to do it myself. Unfortunately, I didn't do it well enough so a young nurse took over and finished the job while I looked away and held my breath in light of the south-of-the-border work area involved. "I should have done a better job huh," I finally said to her.

"Oh that's OK, I do this everyday," she answered as she deftly applied the razor.

Each lab technician came over and introduced his or her self which was a nice touch so typical of St. Joseph's. Each had a specific job to do and told me what it was. They were all very pleasant and did their very best to keep me calm.

One technician was great at reducing the stress level in the room. He was the guy who ran the camera which was going to take the high speed X-ray pictures of my heart. He was positioned behind a glass wall near a computer screen. He had a microphone and could speak to the whole crowd when he needed to. First thing he said was, "Hello Robert.

Your last name is Benson correct?"

"Yes," I called out dutifully.

"And you're here for that sex change operation?"

Well the whole team, including me, were laughing at this wonderful ice breaker. I was a happy part of a cheerful bunch of folks about to do a terrific job on my heart.

Enter Dr. William M. Lieppe (pronounced lippy). I know he's a fine doctor who does about 45 of these procedures a week, but I immediately saw the man as more of a fighter pilot, a true top gun. He owned the room when he walked in. The quintessential take charge guy. He sipped his coffee and sat at a little desk to the side of the room as he went over my chart. It was like he was in the mission briefing room on the aircraft carrier Nimitz. Dr. Lieppe was a professional.

He came over, fixed me with his steady, ice blue eyes, introduced himself and told me we were about to begin. I didn't know it at the time but he had already been out in the family room to introduce himself to Amy and my folks. He busted my chops a little about the Yankees hat. I told him I hoped he hadn't gone to medical school at Johns Hopkins University in Baltimore, Maryland seeing that the Yankees had just knocked the Baltimore Orioles out of a trip to the World Series. He shook his head no and told me that since I had the guts to wear that hat into the cath lab I could keep it on during the procedure.

"You get this thing fixed and the hat is yours!" I said, trying to give him some added incentive.

So there we were, God and I; with me on the cath table wearing my Yankees baseball cap ready for whatever was to come.

By then I think I was hooked up to every machine and monitor in the room. There was an IV sending some calming drug through my blood stream and Dr. Lieppe said I would feel a little pin prick. He then took a needle that looked the size of a bayonet and stuck it in my inner, upper right thigh next to the femoral artery. The femoral artery would be the beginning of his pathway to my heart. The needle was to numb the area so he could insert a sheath at the entrance point and then a thin tubular instrument called a catheter. After he pulled the needle out of my thigh he waited a minute or so for the area to become numb and then he inserted a wire into my femoral artery.

He threaded the wire up the femoral artery, through the aorta and into the coronary artery of my heart. Lieppe steered the wire through that trip and magically avoided punching a hole in any of those major vessels and causing a massive hemorrhage.

Pushed along this guide wire, a catheter was inserted that followed the wire into my heart. There I was, wide awake watching the screen to my left and there, clear as day, is this wire in my heart.

Luckily there are no nerves in your heart or arteries, so I couldn't feel a thing. I could see it plain as day, but I couldn't feel it.

Lieppe announced, "We're in." Maybe I've seen too many movies but at that instant he sounded like a veteran submarine skipper who had just guided his U-boat through the anti-submarine nets and into an enemy harbor.

"We're in?"

"Right, take a look." He moved the wire back and forth and there was this strand of metal on the screen moving inside my heart!

"Now let's pump in some thallium solution and see what we've got. We're looking for any blockage that may have caused your attack," said Dr. Lieppe.

Thallium is a liquid that will flow through the vessels of the heart, and it shows up on an X-ray. It reveals where the blood is going and where it's not going. Blood alone does not show up on an X-ray.

Doctor Lieppe pushed on the end of a syringe that had been rigged up to the catheter and the thallium went directly to my heart giving me a strange warm rush all the way down to my waist. This was the day for strange feelings.

As the thallium entered my heart, my buddy behind the computer, Mr. Sex Change, cranked up his high-speed x-ray camera that looked like a big wide telescope. It made a whirring sound while it took pictures in such rapid succession that I could see the thallium move through the heart and the arteries. With each heartbeat I saw the movement of the thallium. The camera began to move side to side and up and down, changing angles and perspective as it searched for the blockage.

Suddenly, Top Gun Lieppe says, "There it is,"

I look at the screen and I don't see anything unusual.

"Where?"

"Right there," he said, pointing to an artery on the screen that looked about as wide as a soda straw on each end but in the middle was crimped down barely to a thread. The artery looked like a small sausage that someone twisted in the middle leaving two links. The thallium was hardly getting through the blockage.

"What is blocking the artery?" I asked.

"Plaque," answered Dr. Lieppe as he stared at the screen. "Usually it forms most readily when there's a high level of cholesterol in the blood. It's really a kind of lump that forms under the innermost layer of the artery. If it grows enough over time, it can cause a blockage like the one you're looking at."

CHAPTER 10

The doctor asked a nurse to go out and tell my family he was going to perform the angioplasty procedure.

"Oh wonderful," I said to myself sarcastically. Amy, Mom and Dad are going to love this news. Actually, however, upon hearing it, my father hugged Amy and told her it was great news. He reasoned that it was wonderful they found the problem and could do something to fix it. He said it would be terrible to know I had a heart attack but not know how or why it happened, and have to live in fear that the defect was buried somewhere ready to cause more serious difficulties in the future.

Back in the lab, Dr. Lieppe inserted a tiny angioplasty balloon into the catheter and ran it up to my heart. With some more of his legerdemain he worked it gently into my left anterior descending artery where the blockage was located. Up to that point I didn't know I had a left descending anterior artery but as blood vessels go, your left anterior descending is a major one. If you picture Manhattan as the heart, then Broadway is the left anterior descending artery. I think it helps feed blood to the lungs which may explain my heavy breathing during tennis.

Dr. Top Gun then rigged in a relatively new piece of equipment called a stent. It's a small latticed metal cylinder that encircles the tiny balloon. It looks pretty much like one of those little springs you find inside some ball point pens that you click to expose the point.

When he got it in place, he inflated the balloon causing this mechanism to expand the stent to form a type of tunnel support in the artery.

After he put in two of these stents at the blockage point, he told me they should help keep the artery open wide enough to allow the blood to flow through freely.

The balloon inflation part of the procedure got my full attention. When the little balloon was expanded it cut off the blood flow, giving me the same pressure feeling I had at the mail box. Because Top Gun was in the target area, he wanted to take full advantage of the opportunity and do the job right. He wanted to give me the maximum opening he could safely give me so he left the balloon open for what felt like two days. It was really only about 15 seconds. He told me that because I'm young and enjoy strong arterial walls he could use sufficient inflation to assure an open artery. It felt like an elephant was standing on one foot, squarely in the center of my chest. As he expanded the balloon, I casually mentioned,

"Doc, Doc, Doc!"

He said, "Two more seconds," and then deflated and retracted the balloon. What a glorious feeling it was as the blood flowed through again. Something like coming up for air after you've stayed under water too long.

Dr. Lieppe got up and announced, "We're done."

Mr. Sex Change printed a before and after picture of the clogged artery for the doctor and made a copy for me. As they unhooked me from all the equipment, the doctor showed me the pictures. He seemed to be very pleased with them and said it was quite dramatic! "What does that mean?," I asked myself.

It meant that while the actual damage to my heart, if any, was very minor, the blockage itself was anything but minor. Playing tennis with my artery in that blocked condition was like closing the Los Angles Freeway during rush hour. If I had ignored that message at the mail box, sooner rather than later my heart would have seized up and failed.

Mr. Sex Change helped me off the table, which

was a bit of a chore in that he had to guard the wound in my leg where the catheter had been inserted. As he gently wrestled me off the table I found my face buried in his armpit.

"Hmmmm, lovely. Is that Mennen Roll On?" I inquired.

"You're just lucky you caught me early in the morning," he replied.

I really loved that guy.

I handed the Yankee cap to Dr. Lieppe and told him it was his. He took it but put it back on my head and said, " No, you keep it. It's your lucky hat now."

With that he went off to show the pictures to some of his colleagues. They wheeled me out to the hall outside the lab and my family was there beaming and happy to see me. Lieppe had given them the good news.

The balance of the day was for rest and reliving my experience in the lab. The procedure had shocked my system enough to make me feel a little weak and not quite ready to leap tall buildings in a single bound. Overall, I felt relieved and pretty good. My mind told me that I made it, I survived, but it also started to come up with the nagging questions of why it had happened and how do I prevent it from happening again and whether I was prone to having plaque build up in my arteries.

Dr. Margolis was going to work with me on those

questions but he wouldn't be able to change my life. God willing, I would be able to do that myself. As it turned out, Dr. Margolis was as good at the non-invasive aspects of my treatment as Dr. Lieppe was in the lab. He was like the understanding gymnastics coach who helps you over the fear of falling. He gently rebuilt my confidence. He told me what to expect so when the feelings of sadness and lack of worth began to hit me I better understood them. I was motivated to please him as I faced the diet and exercise phases of my recovery and, like a kid, I was tickled pink when he complimented my progress.

CHAPTER 11

While I was recovering at St. Joseph's, friends and neighbors came by to see how I was doing. I was starting to understand why God didn't give us a perfect world. I'm no philosopher, but it stands to reason that if we had a perfect world with no sickness, hardship or need, then there would be little or no opportunity for us to be loving, caring or charitable. A simple visit to the hospital does wonderful things to both the visited and the visitor. Come to think of it, I did my friends and neighbors a great service by giving them a chance to visit me at St. Joseph's. Of course I'm kidding. I was humbled by their kindness and I can't tell you how great it made me feel to crack jokes and just sit and chat about everyday happenings with our friends. They were terrific.

It became apparent that many of the questions asked by my male friends about my experience were calculated to help them ease their own minds about whether they also were candidates for a heart attack. Each kept trying to place himself in a category other than mine. I didn't give them much solace.

"This must run in your family, right?" It doesn't.

"You had high blood pressure, I guess?" Not at any level near what you would associate with a heart attack.

"Your cholesterol must have really been up there?" A little high but not sky high.

"Were you ever a smoker?" No.

"You probably had chest pains before, right?" Nope.

"Did you see it coming?" No way.

Most of my friends probably participated to some extent in the same kind of rat race as I did but they didn't seem to suspect that the stresses and strains of it, unless managed, could take a toll on their physical wellbeing. Why should they? I never thought of it either.

The next day, Tuesday, was more rest and visits from friends and family. My folks brought me a St. Joseph medal to wear. St. Joseph is the patron saint of the working man and he was the head of a pretty important family. That plus the fact that the hospital was named for him made the medal very appropriate.

There was a note with it that read, "Here's a St. Joseph medal. You do the work and let him do the worrying."

Some calls from friends came in and a couple from co-workers. I had alerted them that I would be away from the job for a while. One of the calls was from the President of our division. The other was from my boss. I was grateful that they picked up the phone to call me.

I used to pride myself in being the youngest guy present in important business meetings. On Tuesday, I got rolled around the cardiac unit in a wheelchair to give me a break from the small hospital room. I quickly realized that I was the youngest patient there as well.

Tuesday also was a day for meeting with the post-operative teams which are supplied by the hospital. The titles of the members of the teams tipped me off on the issues I had to address to ward off another attack. There was a dietary advisor, cardiac rehabilitation advisor and a stress management advisor. Amy and I conversed with each of them and they signed me up and scheduled future sessions. I began to see what it was going to take to get my strength back and the changes I had to make in my life. Toward the end of the day, I was told that tomorrow, I would be going home.

I spent the rest of the evening thanking every hospital nurse or other staff member I saw for the way I had been treated. The people at St. Joseph's sincerely care about every sick person that walks or rolls through their door.

I still wonder what would have happened to me if I had gone to some HMO that was motivated by both care and cutting costs. Mine was one of those very close cases where the decision to keep me or send me hung by a thread. It would be silly to think that a cost cutting motivation would not have altered that critical call. If you tell a home plate umpire that he has to drastically speed up the game, it will broaden his strike zone. Thank you, God, for every person that dealt with me at St. Joseph's and put my life ahead of the profit of some insurance company.

CHAPTER 12

My last night in St. Joseph's I received a telephone call from Dr. Sergio Fashetti (not his real name). Sergio is a friend of my father and Dad asked him to call me to talk about stress and how to handle it.

Dr. Fashetti holds four doctorate degrees: theology, psychology, philosophy and medicine. Born and raised in Italy, his accent is charming and adds spice to his wisdom.

I picked up the phone.

"Bob, we have never met. I am Sergio Fashetti."

"Hi Doctor, how are you?"

"I am well thank you. How are you doing?"

I filled him in and he assured me that I was lucky to have some of the best doctors available looking after me.

"Your father tells me you may have some stress in your life," he said.

I told him that before the heart attack, I never gave much thought to stress but I knew I was always on the run to the point that if my hair were on fire I probably would have kept running rather than take the time to put it out.

"And your eating habits were deplorable, I would venture."

"I'm a fast food junkie," I admitted. "I seldom have time for a regular sit down meal."

"I hope you mean you <u>were</u> a fast food junkie," Sergio responded. "It is your father's Anglo-Saxon work ethic that has you in trouble. You must become more Italian like me, including the substitution of a little olive oil for the butter or other fats you cannot tolerate. Eating a meal should involve less stuffing and more tasting."

I heard him chuckle softly on the other end of the line.

"What do I do about the stress, given that I'm not lucky enough to be Italian?" I asked.

"It is not the stress that is dangerous," he answered. "It is the anger, especially pent up anger."

"I'm not sure I follow you."

"We all have stress in our lives, it cannot be avoided. It is our reaction to the stress that is critical. If the reaction is to get angry, over time it can be very destructive. Some vent anger and others were raised to be polite so they keep it inside. Either way, anger can lead to a number of health problems including heart attacks. A good sense of humor can help. Let me digress a moment to tell you a story that happened while I was in medical school.

"I had two classmates who had a rather unique method of handling the stresses that abound in medical training. They took every opportunity to embarrass each other in public. They were fast friends and shared great affection for the other, nevertheless, they continually trapped each other in good natured public ridicule. I'll call them Smith and Jones.

"We were in class one morning listening to a very poorly delivered lecture in obstetrics. Smith and Jones were sitting together and Smith fell asleep. In a few moments he started snoring loudly, to Jones great pleasure. Jones made no attempt to disturb his repose.

"Hearing the snoring, the professor focused on Smith and called upon him to recite. Jones gave Smith the elbow and Smith, still groggy, got to his feet.

" 'Have you been following our discussion?" asked the professor.

" 'Yes sir," lied Smith.

" 'Good. We have been covering the methods of delivery of a newborn, Mr. Smith. How many such methods are there?"

Smith glanced down at Jones with a panic stricken 'help me' look.

Jones, his head down, whispered, "Three," and Smith automatically relayed that answer to the professor.

" ' Would you be kind enough to name them for us?' " queried the professor.

"Well of course there is the normal vaginal delivery. Then there is the Cesarean section and of course the....."

Jones whispered, "Anal."

"The anal delivery," said Smith to the professor and he wished immediately that he could retract those words. He had been had and the whole class knew it.

The professor was in seventh heaven. How often did he have such an opportunity to pin a smart aleck to the wall. "Ah yes, Mr. Smith. The child is delivered through the anus. We would all be indebted to you if you would describe the anal delivery for us."

"I would be most happy to sir," replied Smith, "but it would be much more instructive if Mr. Jones here would describe it since he himself was born that way."

Sergio then gave me one of his methods for avoiding having anger corrode your health, he said, "LET THEM WIN."

After we hung up, I pondered what in the world he

meant by that. How could I just let them win? I wasn't being paid by my employer to take a dive and not fight to have the company excel. Rolling over would be more stressful to me than the struggle to win. Then it dawned on me. Sergio was telling me that in all those minor contests that go on every day, if they win, let them win. Let those irritating losses go and move on to something else.

I've been in situations where my flight was canceled at the last minute but I wasn't willing to accept it. I would go to the counter and instead of working on alternate travel, I would waste time condemning the airline, dredging up their past failures, fuming and feeling sorry for myself. I should have let them win. They weren't going to uncancel the flight so what was the point of useless post mortems.

Lou Holtz, the former Notre Dame head football and current head football coach of the University of South Carolina, uses the acronym W.I.N. as good advice on handling adversity. The letters stand for, "What's Important Now?". When something bad happens to you, ask yourself what is important now. Take those necessary positive steps, let go and move on.

CHAPTER 13

Morning came and Amy came to pick me up. I was up early to shower, shave and get all the wires and needles out and off of me. The most pain I felt the whole time I was in the hospital was when they jerked the tape that was holding my IV in place off my arm. I'm a hairy rascal in certain places and that tape can be murder.

Dr. Margolis saw me before we departed and said, "all's well that ends well."

I learned that God had to pull some strings to get Basil Margolis to me. Basil was born of Jewish parents and raised in Zimbabwe of all places and then educated in London. Somehow, God got him from those far off places to Atlanta to be on duty at St. Joe's, a Catholic hospital, when I needed him. His accent sounds British. He has the calm aura about him that would make him perfect for talking disturbed people off the ledges of tall buildings if he weren't otherwise engaged in saving lives.

A hospital candy striper wheeled me out to the entrance of the hospital. While I was waiting for Amy to bring the car around, I got talking to a chubby guy, who looked to be in his fifties, as best as I could tell because he was wearing a kind of surgical mask. He asked why I was in the hospital. I told him and then I nodded, "I know, I know," when he told me I was too young. He told me he had had a heart replacement two months before.

"Wow," I offered and asked him how he was doing.

He said the donor had been a fourteen-year-old boy and it was causing him a problem.

"What's that," I said.

"I have this uncanny urge to chase cheerleaders again." He laughed, patted me on the shoulder, turned and went on his way. I loved that guy, too.

Amy drove me home slower than usual, as if she were transporting a fragile vase. We commented on what a great day it was. A beautiful fall day. Sun's out and clear blue skies. I told Amy that my one goal for the day was to get to the bus stop to meet the kids as they got home from school. Amy reminded me that a trip to the bus stop would fit neatly into my exercise schedule which was to walk everyday for 10 minutes the first week and then gradually increase the time thereafter.

Two-thirty arrived. I was pumped to go to the bus stop. Off we went but after a few steps I was starting to drag. When I got halfway there I was wondering if I would make it. The bus stop is only 200 yards from our front door! This coming from a guy who felt like he could lift a car five days before. I got to the bus stop and I was pooped.

A neighbor close to the bus stop ran and got a lawn chair so I could sit and wait for the bus. I sat there dreading the 200-yard forced march back to the house. Maybe Amy could go get the car. Sounds funny, but I was totally bushed. The kids arrived and I got hugs from our own and from some of the neighborhood children. Some of them gave me get well cards they drew on the bus. Pretty wonderful, little K-5 graders thought enough to draw and sign a card for me on the way home from school. One little boy put a dollar in his card because he thought it would make it extra special. Another boy, the son of the woman who ran and got me the chair, prepared one early in the morning when he got himself dressed. He had on an East Carolina University shirt, my alma mater. It was a shirt I had given his Dad. He told his Mom he was going to wear it because Mr. Benson would enjoy seeing it when he got off the bus. What a thoughtful, nice kid! I was getting a taste of the joy in the world outside the rat race.

CHAPTER 14

Let me try to provide a layman's perspective of the medical reasons for my heart attack. Again, my blood pressure was a borderline 140/90. My cholesterol level was a little high. I had no family history of heart attacks. I didn't smoke and my weight was not an issue at 190 pounds because I'm about 6'2". So how come the heart problems?

I had stress that I wasn't managing in the right way. We all have an innate reaction to stressful situations the experts call the "Fight or Flight" reflex. This reflex developed in our ancestors from their reactions to the world around them. To them, life provided almost daily situations in which they had to fight or run for their lives. Modern-day man faces different kinds of stresses, but his body chemistry in reacting to these stresses mirrors that of his ancestors.

Problem is that modern man doesn't usually take the physical action to utilize the fight or flight adrenaline that gets pumped into the blood.

As I understand it, the adrenaline forces the liver to produce cholesterol in anticipation of the need for it to fortify the body for the upcoming fight or flight.

Cholesterol is carried in the blood bound to protein particles. There are two types of particles, HDLs and LDLs. The LDLs take the cholesterol to the tissues where it is needed but if it reaches excess levels it begins to carry it into artery linings to form plaque. HDLs, called good cholesterol, transport excess LDL back to the liver for disposal so that it reduces the chances of a build up of plaque.

Our ancestors used up the cholesterol better than we do. I'm sure this is a gross simplification but it was my habit of internalizing stress and turning it into anger that caused the trouble. I imagine it started something like this:

My great, great, great.......great grandfather lived eons ago somewhere in what is now called Scandinavia. His mother named him Benk. In her later stages of pregnancy with him, she enjoyed sitting at the mouth of their cave when it rained and listening to the drops of water splash down on a flat rock. It made the sound, "Benk, benk, benk, benk." That was the rhythm of her music. Some of the birds provided the melody. She had no Elton John CD's to listen to.

One morning after he reached manhood, Benk walked out of the cave and inhaled the fresh, misty morning air. It was refreshing after the smoky stillness inside. Benk began sniffing the air for the scent of game as he hoisted and balanced his spear. For that time, his spear was technologically advanced because its tip was fashioned out of a primitive bronze.

Now Benk was ready to go to work. He was a hunter.

Following scent and spoor, he began tracking a small boar into a narrow valley and just when he thought he had it cornered, he heard the basso grunt of a large cave bear. With that, the bear rose on its hind legs out of a growth of large ferns not ten yards in front of him.

Benk's brain and body immediately reacted to cope with the situation. As he quickly considered whether to attack the bear or run from it, his heart beat faster, his blood pressure rose and his other body systems acted to alter the chemistry of his blood.

Benk took physical action. My guess is that he attacked and killed the bear after a terrific struggle but in any event, after taking the strenuous physical action, his body systems returned to normal.

Benk had a son, whom he called "Benkson". Centuries later, they dropped the "k" so they called me Benson.

Grandpa Benk caused me a problem. I inherited his body system's tendency to quickly react to stressors. Of course, no cave bears had challenged me lately but I did have those other predicaments such as canceled flights, computers down, traffic jams, quotas, late shipments, canceled orders and the like. My system reacted much as Benk's did when he saw the bear but, unlike him, I took no physical action to trigger a return of my system to normal. I simply sat and stewed and that was dangerous to my health. The formation of the plaque that blocked my artery was abetted by my reaction to stress and it was something I had to address in order to ward off another attack.

CHAPTER 15

To drive home the point that emotions and handling stress can have a direct effect on body chemistry and functions, consider the following kinds of statements that we hear every day. In each one there is an event that alters the body in different ways and different places:

* * * * *

"Shamus, put the bagpipes away will ya, you're giving me a headache."

"Did you notice how beet-red Wilson's ears got when we questioned him about his September results."

"When Arthur proposed to me back in 1936, I got weak in the knees and threw up."

"I was watching America's Funniest Home Videos. They showed a wedding ceremony and right in the middle of it the groom keeled right over."

"When the boss called me into his office, I broke out in cold sweats."

"Why Helen, you're blushing. You must be very fond of that young man."

"My hands were shaking so badly I could hardly reach out and accept the bowling trophy."

"That Stephen King novel gave me goose bumps."

"Oh my gosh, when I saw that semi coming through the red light I got that strange copper taste in my mouth."

"Normally he doesn't stutter. It's only when he gets upset."

"Mom, I'm calling to give you some news. Are you sitting down?"

"Well sir, when I saw that bloody ice pick, the hair on the back of my neck stood up."

"Jimmy was so cute. He went to the eighth grade dance and danced with Lu Ella Barnes. He said she trembled and his palms got soaking wet."

"I don't know how Phil handled it. When he came out of the delivery room, his face was ashen."

"He got so choked up, he never finished the best man's toast."

"When the jury came back with that guilty verdict. He wet his pants right there at the defense table."

* * * * *

I rest my case.

CHAPTER 16

Little did I know that the road to recovery would be so enlightening. I don't mean the physical aspects of recovery so much, although they were both demanding and humbling. It was the emotional and spiritual aspects of coming back from a heart attack that made me face some of the unpleasant facts about myself.

The physical part of rehabilitation consisted mainly of following orders. I signed up to attend a three-day-per-week class at the hospital. I walked on treadmills, rode a bicycle and worked the armgome-ter, a type of stationary bike for the arms. I met some unforgettable people while I was enrolled in the pro-gram, many of them scared and all of them with more serious ailments than mine.

During class we were hooked up to heart monitors

and the therapists continually checked our vital signs as we went through the workout routine.

The human mind and body are in constant communication with each other. The mind tells the body to stand, sit or climb a tree. The body tells the mind such information as it's in pain, hungry, tired, drowsy, numb or in need of a shot of bourbon. After a heart attack the body tells the mind it is fatigued and wants to curl up in a corner. A big part of the physical therapy involves having the mind ignore and override that feeling to the extent necessary to return to health. It's something like the mind/body battle that a dieter or a recovering alcoholic goes through. It can be upsetting at first because you feel very frail and you fear your heart won't be up to it. It was upsetting for me for a couple of other reasons.

First, I was 36 years old doing exercises with folks that had 30 or more years on me. I began to second guess what I was doing there. I felt like a teenager in a nursing home.

I had a cheerful thought that since we weren't grouped together based on age, maybe we were put together based on life expectancy. I stuck it out because I was ashamed to face my family and tell them I quit.

As time passed, the individuals in our physical therapy class started to form into a kind of team. We supported and cheered each other's tiniest advancement. We got to be friends.

I tried to speak with each of the participants about what happened to them and how they felt. All were heart patients. To my left was a man who had his second round of by-pass surgery. He was frustrated and dejected and argued with the nurses that he needed his protein and he was going to continue to eat steak! His body was winning the battle over his mind. I wanted to help change his mind but there was nothing I could add to the advice he was getting from the nurses.

Straight ahead was a guy who just had his third heart attack. One day he told us about a new home he was building in the Georgia mountains. Unfortunately, he never got to the mountains or his new home. He died two days later. May God be good to him.

Behind me was a fellow for whom I pray daily. He has a new heart. From the way he talked, he spent every waking hour wondering if his body would reject it. Every time his legs moved those stationary bicycle pedals I could read his face as he anticipated the new heart quitting on him. If he could hang in there, so could I.

There were lighter moments in physical rehab. There were quite a few characters in my class. Many used humor to ease the tension. There was one mature, large, spinster of a woman in the class who talked with me to ease the stress. She referred to herself as an "unclaimed treasure." I think she had some sort of a quota of words she had to express each day but she lived alone and tried to use them up on me. She loved music and one day she brought an old cassette tape recorder to class to play some of her favorites from the fifties for me. Her enthusiasm alone made me enjoy it even though the sound was tinny and scratchy.

One day I listened as she lamented the horrors of AIDS and told me of her volunteer work in the homes of people suffering from that disease.

I rode my stationary bike next to hers and as I progressed in the class and got stronger I would be instructed to pedal faster than my senior teammates.

She would say, "I'll tell you what darling, if that bike breaks loose of that stand, your gonna ride right through that wall." She used to also heckle me about the breeze my bike would throw off. The bikes had big fans as front wheels.

My bike mate was a person of considerable bulk and wore a wig that didn't fool anyone. One day she failed to appear and when I asked after her, I learned two things; one, she had finished the course and two, she was a man, a genuine transvestite. I hope her heart remains as healthy as it is kind.

I took four weeks off from work after the attack. Most patients take six weeks, but my event was not as debilitating as most. I learned that about a third of the folks die of their first heart attack. Looking back on it, I probably should have played it on the safe side and taken six.

At first I wasn't worrying about anything but getting back on my feet and healing. But as time passed, I started to think about the job and what I was missing. I wondered what the company was thinking about my absence and whether I would be thought of as damaged goods. Were they going to save my place in the organization? Would they think I couldn't come back and do the job? Lots of crazy things were floating around in my head.

During the time off, I spent loads of it with Amy. We went to the lake and picnicked. We took a lot of walks hand in hand. I also spent more time than ever putting the kids to bed. Reading books with them. Just carrying on conversations to see how things were going at school. Reading those bedtime stories was ceasing to be a chore and I started looking forward to it. I enjoyed the time together and it stopped being a rush job to get over with so I could get back to those few loose ends left from work.

Look at it this way. Would an employer tolerate you going to the office each day but spending the bulk of your time there on your personal affairs? Somehow, I don't think so. Well, turn about is fair play. Why should your spouse and children have to tolerate you being at home but spending the bulk of your time thinking about or doing work?

I think I aced the physical therapy and diet aspects of my come-back. My weight came down as did my body fat, blood pressure, cholesterol and pulse rate. The post-heart attack period for most victims, however, includes post traumatic stress and depression. I was no exception. The good folks at St. Joseph's told me it was coming, which helps, but it can still be terrible. I went through a time of about three months where I felt like the biggest loser, like something was lacking in me as a person. I was different than I was prior to the attack. I wasn't my jolly, high-powered, old self. I didn't look people in the eye when I talked to them as I did prior to the attack. What was this feeling? Why was I feeling this way?

Enter the father of the young man that wore my alma mater's shirt to school that day to surprise me at the bus stop. He and I had numerous conversations about why I was feeling the way I did. My friend was a former Marine who had watched comrades die in combat and he struggled with guilt over being spared. He had to fight his way through it and he helped me to do the same.

Amy's mom was also a great help to me in facing the fear and frailty. I told her that I spent almost every moment wondering if each pain, itch or sensation was the precursor of another heart attack. She had won a battle with breast cancer and she told me that, for a time, she went through the same kind of dreaded anticipation that her cancer would return. She said it just took time for confidence to return and that I would improve as my strength returned. Both Amy's mom and dad were in my corner. They helped me drag my fears out in the open, get the light of day on them and watch them melt.

CHAPTER 17

I believe what happened to me was a miracle. Maybe not the parting of the Red Sea but a miracle never-the-less. The classic definition of a miracle is, in my judgment, much too narrow. It defines a miracle as an event that is a departure from the known laws of nature. Because it is beyond nature, we call it supernatural. I don't think miracles depend at all on our knowledge of the laws of nature. Take a look up at the sky on a clear night and then try to tell me that we have even begun to scratch the surface of knowing the laws of nature. I think that every time we discover a secret of nature we see a new miracle. That's because God has his hand in there.

The sequence of events that got me to the hospital, the treatment I received and the fact that I suffered no discernible heart damage meet my threshold standard for miracles. Six months after my attack a thal-lium scan looked at my heart down to an eighth of an inch and found no damage. They tell me that every attack causes some damage so I may have had some but, if it's there, they can't find it.

I think it is interesting to view my experience from the perspective of a man who may have lived in earlier times, a man searching for miracles. It's fiction of course, but bear with me.

* * * * *

Nearly six months after the crucifixion of Christ, Sam walked out into his fig tree orchard and gazed up into the starry night sky. His farm was less than ten miles from Jerusalem.

Sam was a troubled man. All about him, his neighbors were excited about a new religious movement that was being ignited by the disciples of Christ. They spoke of a loving god and Sam, as was his nature, was skeptical. He was not at all sure of the existence of a god let alone a loving one who would have time for him. When he spoke with some of the new converts, however, they told him they were actually present when miracles were performed. Sam thought that if only he could witness a miracle. He had the following conversation:

Sam: Please God, if you exist, show me a miracle.

God: Well Sam, you're talking with me, will that

do it for you?

Sam: With all due respect sir, you could be a figment of my imagination.

God: OK, how about a nice sunrise tomorrow, or maybe I can open a rosebud for you, or maybe you can watch an egg hatch.

Sam: I don't mean to be picky but those are pretty commonplace. Can't you show me a real humdinger; a real departure from the laws of nature?

God: Give me a minute. Oh, I'm planning one for another fellow. Perhaps we can work a swap. I could transport you forward in time about 2000 years but you would have to suffer a heart attack .....

Sam: That's not what I had in mind I .....

God: Let me finish. You get the heart attack but then I have a neighbor call you on the telephone and offer to lend you a lawn mower.

Sam: What's a lawn mower?

God: A self-propelled device that cuts grass. All you have to do is walk behind it.

Sam: Wow! What's a telephone?

God: You push a few buttons, sit in your living room and talk with people all over the earth.

Sam: Incredible!

God: There's more. The neighbor tells you to go see a doctor so you climb into a chariot that needs no horses, camels, donkeys or anything and it runs on wheels the rims of which are filled with air to cushion the ride.

Sam: You are kidding!

God: Wait. While you are in the chariot, you push a button and listen to a man named Springstein sing a song.

Sam: Is Mr. Springstein in the chariot with me?

God: No. As a matter of fact his song was actually sung in an arena in a place called New Jersey some ten years before and then it was saved so you could listen to it at your leisure.

Sam: How could that be?

God: I thought you wanted miracles.

Sam: Right but what you are describing is pretty overwhelming.

God: Sam, even my children will be able to do this stuff and besides I do some of my best work through mortals. There is more. You get to the doctor and he has someone stick a metal straw in your leg, run it up inside your body to your heart and fix your heart while you watch the whole thing through a kind of electronic window.

Sam: My God!

God: What?

Sam: Sorry, It's just an expression we use. Anyway, where would you find such a doctor?

God: He would come from thousands of miles away on a flying machine that goes six miles high and goes along at about 500 miles per hour. Would all that satisfy your need for a miracle?

Sam: Who wouldn't be satisfied, but to get it I have to have a heart attack?

God: That's the deal. Of course I could keep things as originally planned and you could settle for tomorrow's sunrise.

Sam: Thank you God. I think I'll take the sunrise.

God: Go in peace Sam and don't be a stranger.

* * * * *

I'm sure 2000 years of science has made me more advanced as to the laws of nature than Sam was but I am no less in awe of the things that happened to me. They clearly were miracles to him and are no less to me. I hope I never get so smart that I fail to marvel over both the simple, and the complex wonders of God's love.

I also hope that I never make myself a stranger. On the other hand, I don't want to be a nudzh either. "Nudzh" is the Yiddish word for pest. You know, "Hi God, it's me again. Now about that BMW I asked you for. Just a little bump up on some of my stocks and it's mine. See ya. Gotta run."

You have to figure that if God is infinite and omnipotent and omniscient, he must have a half decent memory. Treat Him as a good friend. Talk with Him often, show respect and love.

How does the Stephen Schwartz song in Godspell

go? "Day by day. Day by day. Oh dear Lord, three things I pray. To see thee more clearly. To love thee more dearly. To follow thee more nearly, day by day." That pretty well sums it up.

CHAPTER 18

The common concept of the rat race is simply a bunch of rats running in a circle without plan or purpose. I picture my rat race as a perpetual merry-go-round that exists in my mind. Hard work and long hours did not create it; it was a matter of attitude. I think that two people may do the same job and expend the same hours doing it, but one can be in the rat race while the other is not. The prevailing attitude of the rat racer is that he is self absorbed in the trappings of the job.

My merry-go-round was very exclusionary. Amy and the kids didn't get to ride. They stood outside the circle and watched me go around and around pretending I was having a wonderful time. They also watched me struggle to get seated on one painted pony after another, each a little closer to the device that dispensed the rings and the occasional gold one that we called a "raise." I was deluded into thinking that my main purpose in life was to throw those rings to my family; to be a good provider. I thought that pretty much exhausted my family obligations.

My family stuck it out better than I deserved. In time, I think the boredom would have gotten to them and they would have wandered away feeling detached and let down regardless of the size of my paycheck. They needed more of my interest and love than I was providing.

A fellow rat racer told me that he once was on a business trip out of town and called home. He spoke with his wife for a while and then asked to speak with his four-year-old daughter. He heard his wife say, "Sandy, Daddy's on the phone and he'd like to talk with you."

Then he heard a small voice answer, "Tell him I'm in a meeting."

AT&T once ran a terrible television ad that touted a picture phone by showing a working mother on a business trip having the pleasure of watching her child being tucked in bed back at home. It almost sounded as if that was as good as being there. Now AT&T is wiser. A current ad shows a working mother (a lawyer) telling her small kids that she can't take them to the beach because she has a meeting with an important client. One of the kids looks up to her and says, "When can I be a client?" The mother takes the kids to the beach where she handles the meeting by using an AT&T cellular phone.

My overused lament was that I wished I had more time for day to day family life. No wonder I had no time. The rat race is a tight circle. It has no beginning and no end. Time, on the other hand, consists of a past, a present and a future. The rat racer remains locked in the present. It's a terrible reiteration of getting up, working and going to bed and no one wins a rat race. Being locked in the present, the rat race becomes as meaningless as listening to only one note of a symphony without reference to the notes played earlier and without anticipation of the notes to follow. It's like trying to get pleasure out of looking at a single frame of the film "The Wizard of Oz."

I wish I could say that I had the sense to jump off my merry-go-round. I simply fell off when I had the heart attack. I did take the opportunity to break the circle and to change my attitude and perspective on life and to stop living solely in the present. Now, I'm trying to see life more as a straight line with a past that is rich in experience and memories; a present where my work is motivated by a desire to help others and a future with loving goals and ambitions for our family. The irony of this change is that I seem to be more effective at work. What was a terrible crisis before is now a little bump in the road of life. Maybe the panic is gone from my eyes, maybe there is less knee-jerk reaction to things and maybe I'm easier to deal with. At the very least, I like myself more.

CHAPTER 19

Every couple has its battles. I'm not talking about physical stuff because if that's going on in your marriage, call time out and get help now. I'm talking about the little verbal zingers aimed at bolstering your own importance and keeping the spouse in line. The rat race provides marvelous targets of opportunity for both participants.

That's because it drives each party into thinking that he or she is alone in many aspects of the marriage.

Here's how I think it works. If I vest my total energy in bringing home a pay check, then I set that paycheck up as a target of opportunity. Sooner or later I am going to try to excuse some negative element of my conduct by pointing to what a great provider I am. The return salvo zeros in on my paycheck because I am waving it aloft like a flag. I would guess something like, "You talk like we're rich. You must be dreaming. Have you ever checked our bank balance at the end of the month?"

I must fire back and I must make the shot count. Now, because I have limited my responsibility to bringing home a paycheck, it becomes my wife's sole responsibility to run the house. I take careful aim and say, "That bank balance would be much healthier if you didn't spend money like it's going out of style."

"Well, if you took some interest in our home you would know that most of the money I spend is to give you a nice place to live."

"I'd settle for a little dusting and picking things up once in a while."

"When's the last time you picked up a broom?"

You get the picture but I think I have a solution. In a battle, one side will hold its fire if its own troops are in the target area. Breaking out of the rat race ends the self absorption. It becomes **our** paycheck, **our** home to furnish and maintain, **our** lawn to mow and **our** problems to work on. The kids' grades at school reflect how well **we** helped them with their homework and how much interest **we** took in their lives. The new focus is on helping each other and caring for each other.

When one of us does well, we all deserve to celebrate. When one of us fails, the others pick us up.

Family teamwork is nothing more than loving each other and showing it by our actions.

When I get home now, I don't rush to the mail and the answering machine. I want my family to know how happy I am to be there.

Never underestimate the importance of a hug. The afternoon I got home from the hospital, my next door neighbor saw me get out of the car and he had learned of my heart attack. He uttered no words but he said plenty when he walked up my driveway, put his arms around me and gave me a hug. I still feel the warmth of it.

When in doubt, err on the side of over-hugging.

CHAPTER 20

I still get angry. I'm working on it but I still get angry. When I think about it I come up with three classes of people that still get to me. As to them, I'm very much a work in progress. They are the dishonest, the arrogant and the people who just don't care.

How do you deal with a person that you believe to be dishonest? There can be no trust certainly. Respect goes out the window.

My theory is that most of us strive for the truth. As kids we ask "Why?" so often that we drive our parents bonkers. We tear open our toys to see the truth about what makes them work. We want people to tell it like it is.

Dishonesty corrupts the search for truth. When I'm in discussions with a person and he tries to add emphasis by saying, "Bob, I'll be honest with you. This is a deal that's good for both of us," I bridle. Maybe it's just an expression but I want to say, "What do you mean you want to be honest with me? What have you been up to this point?"

Now I try to make sure that if I don't believe something I say so. If the person is a habitual liar, I give him the cobra-in-the-cage treatment. If you are in a cage with a cobra, it makes no sense to be angry at the cobra. You protect yourself by understanding that the cobra will never be anything but a cobra and sooner or later he will act like one no matter how hard you work on developing a relationship with him. You don't trust him and you keep your distance but don't eat yourself up being angry at him.

The arrogant also get to me but not nearly as badly as they used to. The arrogant take pride in their own self importance while they show contempt for others. Maybe they bug me so much because I might have acted that way myself at times.

We all seek a long, healthy life. My heart attack taught me that in spades. Being angry at those I consider arrogant is counter productive and dangerous to me and threatens my life. I have to become more compassionate toward them and there is a good rational for that compassion.

Arrogant people are running a bluff. They don't really believe they are superior to anyone. They just want to make us think they are. Because they are running a bluff, they are scared to death that they will be found out; that someone will call their hand and the pot will go elsewhere. There is no reason to be angry at someone who's on such shaky ground.

The third category of people who get to me are those who don't seem to care about me or themselves. I used to rush into an auto rental agency at an airport with no time to spare to get to a meeting and the person behind the counter would tell me in an off hand matter that it will be about a thirty-minute wait for a car. My reaction, of course, would be negative, but just how negative would depend on whether the person showed any concern or appreciation for my problem.

If I got a, "Let me call the garage and see if Tony can speed things up for us," that would be one thing. If, on the other hand, I get a blank stare or if she devoted her time to a close examination of her fingernails, that would be something else.

What I would try to do now would be to show some appreciation for her problem. If cars are being held up at the garage, she is probably getting pounded by other irate customers. She would much prefer to have cars available and avoid the pounding. The, "I don't care," attitude may simply be a defense mechanism.

We all want to be loved. Tell her you understand

it's a rough situation for her and you would appreciate anything she could do to help. Ask her if you could help in any way.

It is very hard not to care about someone who seems to care about you as a person. Weigh this approach against threatening to ruin her and her company and then sitting in a corner while the anger eats away at you.

Want to see a face light up? Ask the lady selling tokens in a subway toll booth how she's doing. She waits on thousands of people a day but, in all probability, you will be the only one to show some interest in her as a person.

Notice in the three examples I've described, I mentioned that we are seekers of life, truth and love. Guess where the only pure forms of life, truth and love reside? I'll give you a hint. Think of a three letter word beginning with a capital "G."

CHAPTER 21

A very important aspect of the road to recovery for me was a very regimented nutrition and exercise plan. Although stress was a very big part of my heart attack, I can't ignore the fact that my eating habits were horrendous. I would eat anything, anytime, anyplace. Snack cakes, fast food, bacon, sausage; you name it, I ate it. I would gorge myself with fast food just to get quick relief from a feeling of hunger. I didn't take the time to consider eating responsibly and correctly. Casual dining is not a rat race activity.

I learned very quickly that along with the other changes I needed to make, my eating and exercise habits also had to change. At the hospital, I met with a nutritionist who explained the dos and don'ts of eating correctly. I committed myself to her program. I also made up my mind to do the exercise necessary to get in better shape. Most of these things were just common sense but I had ignored them before the attack.

Let me emphasize that what I embarked upon in my dietary changes was not a diet. To me, going on a diet means a temporary change in eating habits. What I did and what made the difference for me was a lifestyle change. I not only changed what I was eating, I also modified when I ate and how fast I did it. I began to enjoy the taste of things like the flavor of a single grape. I noticed the texture of food and the aroma surrounding it.

My primary goal was to rid my body of excess fat and to train my heart to be a very healthy and efficient muscle. I didn't want it to be working as hard as it had been. For that reason, I watched my fat intake like a hawk. There are all kinds of guides as to how many grams of fat should be taken in on a daily basis. I don't think it's the same for everyone. I received counseling at the hospital where they took me through a risk factor assessment class to determine my individual fat gram intake levels. I opted to keep my fat intake very low at first until I achieved my weight-loss goal. Consequently, I limited myself to a daily total of only 7-11 grams of fat until my weight dropped to 170 pounds.

I am not a doctor and I don't mean to suggest my

approach to anyone but it did work for me and results came fairly quickly. I never cheated on myself. I followed my own rules without wavering. I started losing the spare tire around my middle. The last excess fat to disappear were those love handles we love to joke about. When mine came off, I felt as if I wasn't loaded with extra baggage any longer. My body fat percentage went from 15% down to 9%.

The foods I stuck to are as follows:

Breakfast: cereal, skim milk, cut up fruit in the cereal, bagel with jam but no butter, juice, pancakes (light syrup and no butter), non-fat yogurt.

Lunch: Turkey or very lean ham sandwiches, mustard, non-fat cheese, lettuce, tomato, pickles, diet soda, juices, tuna, non-fat mayonnaise and relish.

Dinner: Chicken, turkey burgers, veggie burgers, pork tenderloin, pasta, marinara sauce, shrimp, broiled or grilled fish and steamed vegetables.

Snacks: Pretzels, carrot sticks, celery, non-fat cookies. Red wine.

I should mention that I didn't skip a meal. Before my heart attack I used to skip breakfast because I felt I didn't have time. I would grab a coke and off I would go. Now I find that once I started eating breakfast, I don't need to eat as much for lunch. Eating breakfast was another one of those helpful changes in accomplishing my goals.

Low fat foods such as the ones I mentioned above

may sound pretty boring but I wasn't looking for the excitement of another heart attack.

After I met my weight goal of 170 pounds, I started to add fat grams. I now stay around 25-40 grams a day. The body needs some fat, it's the excess that gets you. I don't worry about calories, just fat. That's because I also have a rigorous regimen of exercise as part of my lifestyle change.

It's interesting the way some of these changes have attracted other people to do the same. For example, at many meetings and conferences I attend, during the afternoon breaks they roll out fat-heavy cookies and ice cream. I changed that at some of those sessions by ordering raw vegetables, pretzels and fruit. It gets eaten, I get no complaints and many tell me they think it's a good idea. Maybe adults would feel awkward complaining that they didn't get their cookie but I think I'm doing the right thing. In addition, when eating out, my dining partners often confer with me before they order. They know I'm eating low fat and healthy and they sometimes take cues from me. I think it's great. Whatever I can do to help.

The Cardiac Rehabilitation Center at St. Joseph's configured a nifty exercise routine for me. I started out walking, then went into a jog/walk routine and finally worked up to a full run. They knew what they were doing and I'm pleased with the results. They taught me the importance of warming up for exercise. When I go to the gym now, I'm astounded at how so many people shock their bodies into an exercise routine. It is important to stretch, warm up, work out and then cool down.

Without fail, I run each and every day for twenty minutes. I start out slowly and then work my way up to the point where my heart is at 75% of the maximum range for my age. I wear a device on my wrist that gives me that measurement. I understand that exercise longer than twenty minutes has diminishing returns with regard to cardiovascular benefits. Longer exercise routines do build stamina, however.

I know that the subject of healthy heating and exercise makes some peoples' eyes glaze over. I've become hooked on the subject because of my heart attack. I was pretty dumb to wait. Maybe you don't have plaque building up in your arteries. Then again, maybe you do. How about some preventive maintenance?

I can report that as the result of the program I took on, all of the vital signs- blood pressure, weight, heart rate, body fat percentage, body tone and cholesterol levels have markedly improved. I don't apologize for being proud of that.

CHAPTER 22

I've always believed that we fight our most important battles within ourselves. Before my heart attack, I saw my internal struggle as being one between ambition and patience. At work, I spent a good deal of my time impatiently awaiting the next "atta boy," the next raise or the next promotion. I would grow more impatient when any of those goodies went to someone else.

I viewed ambition as a vital quality to possess. I told myself that I would never get ahead without it. To me, the failures in life were those poor souls who just didn't have enough ambition.

During my recovery, however, I took the time to look up the word "ambition" and I found it to have revealing origins. It comes from the Latin word "ambitio" which means "to go around." It was the term used to describe the Roman candidates for office who went around among the populace seeking praise, flattery and votes. It's a word that marks a strong desire for power, fame and the ability to distinguish one's self as being more worthy than others.

Consequently, ambition fuels the rat race that has you running in circles and leaves you with that empty, gnawing feeling that comes with never being satisfied with yourself or your accomplishments.

I made up my mind that success in life, and the joy that comes from finding it, depend not on what I get but what I give. That's not a new idea and I'm ashamed that it took me so long to embrace it. It's important to like yourself but you will like yourself more if you think about yourself less. Ambition does not align well with what I believe to be the purpose of my being here on earth. I was put here to love and to help and that's what brings real satisfaction.

I've never met Paul Newman, but my instincts tell me that if you were to ask him whether his success as an actor and the celebrity that has earned for him gives him as much satisfaction as his charity work on behalf of kids, he would think you were a real Bozo. Obviously, giving and filling a need does more for the soul than public adoration and praise can ever do.

Think about the folks in your neighborhood or at work that are doing significant things to help others and I'll bet you dimes-to-doughnuts they are a happy bunch of people - a joy to be around. Unfortunately, there aren't enough of them.

In my neighborhood lives a couple with three children - one in college, another in high school and one in elementary school. Out of love they have taken on the role of foster parents to infants of drug-addicted parents or kids who may have been mistreated or abused. They take in children of all races and make a special loving home for them until the kids can be placed in a healthy permanent situation. I'm impressed by the fact that they are motivated solely by the belief that these kids need them. For the duration of their stay, the children are part of the family where they witness the powers of love, kindness and respect. These people are a joy to be around because they are happy in their giving.

Another neighbor has taken it upon himself to help feed the poor. Often when I drive by his home, I see him tying down huge boxes of fruit, vegetables and other food items to the roof of his small station wagon. He made a deal with a large, local grocer for items that are perfectly good but nearing the end of their shelf life and he transports them to an urban soup kitchen that provides meals for the needy. I feel good watching him load up. Imagine how great he must feel inside.

My favorite example of the joy of helping others is my wife, Amy. It is no accident that good things happen around Amy. I wish I were as quick to sense a need and do something about it as she is. Just being around her makes me proud. I'd like to be more like her.

Amy is the Pied Piper of the kind hearted. Each year she sees to it that we adopt a family to assure they have a magnificent Christmas. She's carried this tradition from our old neighborhood in Winston-Salem, North Carolina, to our current one near Atlanta. She mobilized the entire neighborhood to share in bringing joy to a working couple with five children whose lives are a constant struggle to make ends meet. Amy and her friends talk with the couple to assess their needs and to find out what their kids are asking of Santa. The lists are spread across the neighborhood and poof—the treasure starts flowing in. I have to empty one side of our garage to accommodate it all, each package tagged for a specific member of the family filling a specific need or matching an item on a wish list. One year, St. Ann's Church in Marietta and its parishioners donated five brand new bikes, one for each of the kids. What fun it was to roll them into that tiny home of theirs on Christmas Eve while the kids were off visiting with an aunt.

After we drop off the gifts, I think of the parents sorting them out for the kids and what joy they shared in anticipation of Christmas morning. I was also impressed with the dignity of the dad in accepting what we offered. I wondered, if I were in his shoes would I have allowed my selfish sense of pride to get in the way and gone thumbs down on the gifts. I learned from the guy. As he pitched in to help us unload, he radiated joy and gratitude. Plainly, his kids came first and they were what mattered. He was doing his best for them and it took strength for him to do it. My guess is that he thought no less of himself— he just thought of himself less.

Amy doesn't think her continuous efforts on behalf of others merit any plaudits. It makes her happy to do it. There is a wonderful innocence about her when it comes filling a need, especially where kids are involved. Her parents are both retired teachers and Amy followed in their footsteps. She chose a profession that finds its rewards in helping and nurturing and she chose a life that does the same.

Early in our marriage, I would refuse to go with Amy to deliver the gifts to an adopted family at Christmas. I didn't go because I didn't feel comfortable with the idea of giving at what I thought was the receiver's expense. Amy kept after me and finally I went along. I'm coming around. I'm finding that the joy is in the giving and if the person on the receiving end of the gift also feels good about it then that's an added bonus.

CHAPTER 23

I hope this book will be of some help. My guess is that there are many folks out there with plaque building in their arteries who are helping the process along with fat loaded diets and no exercise. If that's not you, then maybe you are married to one. I also would venture that, like me, many have never thought about handling stress in this complex world of ours. Please see a good doctor and find out where you stand. I thought a heart attack wouldn't happen to me until the twilight of a long life. I was wrong, but I was very lucky. Please don't sluff-off your own good intuitions.

I realize that I stressed my belief in God and his hand in my experience. I'm not planning to start a new sect or sell prayer cloths and I didn't want to be preachy. My intention was simply to deliver an honest account of how I felt. I know God was part of things.

Take the time to slow down long enough to see if you're running 100MPH With Your Hair On Fire.

Peace

Printed in the United States
1220300001B/88-138